THE ART OF TAKING RISK

Welcome and Embrace Challenges, Foster Resilience,
Unlock Doors of Opportunities, and Turn Obstacles
into Triumph.

PRADIP DAS

are declared or implied. Readers acknowledge that the author is not engaging in the rendering of legal, financial, medical or professional advice. The content within this book has been derived from various sources. Please consult a licensed professional before attempting any techniques outlined in this book.

By reading this document, the reader agrees that under no circumstances is the author responsible for any losses, direct or indirect, which are incurred as a result of the use of information contained within this document, including, but not limited to, — errors, omissions, or inaccuracies.

Please see the Author Profile

Table of Contents

Introduction

In my fifty years of life, I've faced numerous challenges and taken risks, often without knowing how things would turn out. Many of these risks played a significant role in shaping my career and future. Interestingly, most of these risks weren't initially chosen by me; they were a result of circumstances. However, when I willingly accepted these challenges, I discovered that those risks ultimately led me to success.

Steve Jobs is someone who took risks and ultimately succeeded. After dropping out of college, Jobs co-founded Apple Computer in his garage with Steve Wozniak. Despite facing setbacks, such as being fired from his own company, Jobs continued to take risks, ultimately leading to the development of products such as the iPod, iPhone, and iPad, which revolutionized the tech industry.

Elon Musk is known for his risk-taking and innovative ideas. He co-founded PayPal, which revolutionized online payments, and went on to found several other successful companies, including SpaceX, Tesla, and The Boring Company. Musk's ideas have been met with skepticism and criticism, but his determination and willingness to take risks have helped him to achieve great success.

J.K. Rowling is another example of someone who took risks and overcame adversity. Before becoming a successful author, Rowling faced numerous rejections from publishers for her Harry Potter series. However, she persisted, self-published the first book, and eventually landed a publishing deal. Her series went on to become a worldwide phenomenon, inspiring a generation of young readers.

Malala Yousafzai is a Pakistani activist who stood up for girls' education, even in the face of Taliban violence. In 2012, she was shot in the head by a Taliban gunman but survived and continued to speak out for education and women's rights. Her bravery and willingness to take risks inspired people around the world, and in 2014, she became the youngest person to receive the Nobel Peace Prize.

Throughout history, great achievements have often been the result of taking risks. From exploring new frontiers to starting a new business, taking risks has been the key to progress and success. However, the very thought of taking risks can be daunting and can cause fear and anxiety for many people. But the truth is, without taking risks, we can never truly know what we are capable of, nor can we achieve our full potential. In this fast-paced and constantly changing world, the ability to take risks and adapt to new challenges is more important than ever. So, what does it mean to take risks? And how can we learn to Accept risk-taking as an essential part of personal and professional growth? In this essay, we will explore the importance of taking risks, the benefits and drawbacks of risk-taking, and strategies for effectively managing and maximizing the impact of risk-taking.

Risk-taking is a fundamental aspect of human nature. It is a fundamental driver of innovation, progress, and success, yet also has the potential to lead to failure, loss, and harm. In today's world, where change is constant, the ability to take risks and adapt to new challenges has never been more important. Whether it is pursuing a new career, starting a new business, or exploring new territories, taking risks is an essential part of personal and professional growth.

However, despite its importance, the very thought of taking risks can be daunting for many people. The fear of failure, uncertainty, and potential consequences can cause anxiety, hesitation, and doubt. But, as with most things in life, success comes to those who are willing to take calculated risks and are not afraid to fail.

What Is Risk Taking?

What does it mean to take risks, and why is it so important? What are the benefits and drawbacks of risk-taking, and how can we effectively manage and maximize the impact of risk-taking in our lives?

Firstly, let's define what we mean by "taking risks." In its simplest form, taking risks means stepping out of one's comfort zone and making a decision that involves some degree of uncertainty, potential danger, or opportunity cost. It could mean investing in a new venture, pursuing a different career path, starting a new relationship, or even skydiving. The degree of risk involved can vary widely, from low-risk decisions with little potential downside to high-risk decisions that could result in significant loss or failure.

Why Taking Risks Is Important

One reason why risk-taking is so important is that it has the potential to lead to significant rewards. In fact, many of the greatest achievements in history were the result of taking calculated risks. For example, the Wright brothers took a massive risk when they attempted to build the first airplane, and their persistence and risk-taking paid off when they achieved the world's first successful powered flight. Similarly, entrepreneurs such as Steve Jobs, Bill Gates, and Jeff Bezos took significant risks when they started their companies, and their innovative thinking and willingness to take chances were essential to their success.

Another reason why risk-taking is important is that it allows us to learn, grow, and develop as individuals. When we take risks, we are forced to step out of our comfort zones and confront new challenges and experiences. This can be daunting, but it also provides an opportunity for personal and professional growth. For example, when we start a new business or pursue a new career path, we are exposed to new ideas, people, and situations, which can help us develop new skills and perspectives.

Significance of risk in personal and professional growth

Risk-taking is a critical component of personal and professional growth. By taking risks, individuals and organizations can challenge themselves, innovate, and ultimately, achieve success.

In personal growth, risk-taking can help individuals overcome fears and limitations, build confidence, and expand their comfort zones. When we take risks, we step out of our familiar routines and try something new, which can lead to personal breakthroughs and transformative experiences. By facing challenges and pushing ourselves beyond our perceived limits, we can grow and develop new skills and talents, broaden our perspectives, and gain valuable life experiences.

In professional growth, risk-taking can help individuals and organizations innovate, grow, and succeed in competitive markets. Successful businesses and entrepreneurs often take calculated risks to differentiate themselves from their competition, develop new products or services, and expand their customer base. By taking risks, organizations can also identify and address potential weaknesses, adapt to changing market conditions, and build resilience.

Of course, taking risks can also lead to failure or setbacks. However, these experiences can provide valuable learning opportunities and help individuals and organizations develop the resilience and adaptability necessary for long-term success. Moreover, by taking risks and learning from failures, individuals and organizations can gain the confidence to tackle bigger challenges and achieve even greater successes.

Overall, risk-taking is a critical ingredient in personal and professional growth. By embracing risk, individuals and organizations can unlock their full potential, innovate, and ultimately, achieve their goals and aspirations.

Risk of Risk Taking

Despite its potential benefits, risk-taking also comes with its fair share of drawbacks. One of the biggest risks of taking risks is the potential for failure. When we take risks, we are exposing ourselves to the possibility of loss, harm, or negative consequences. This can be especially challenging when the stakes are high, such as when starting a new business or pursuing a major career change.

Another drawback of risk-taking is that it can be difficult to manage. While taking risks can be exhilarating and empowering, it can also be overwhelming and cause stress and anxiety. It is important to strike a balance between taking calculated risks and managing the potential downsides.

So, how can we effectively manage and maximize the impact of risk-taking in our lives? The key is to take calculated risks that are aligned with our values, goals, and strengths. This means evaluating the potential risks and rewards of a decision and taking steps to mitigate the potential downsides.

Another strategy for effective risk-taking is to Accept failure as a necessary part of the process. When we take risks, we are bound to experience setbacks and failures.

Impact of Risk Taking in Achieving Success and Happiness

Risk-taking can have a significant impact on achieving success and happiness. Here are some ways in which taking risks can influence our ability to achieve these goals:

Opportunities for Growth: When we take risks, we challenge ourselves to step outside our comfort zones and try something new. This can lead to personal and professional growth, as we develop new skills and experiences. This growth can contribute to our overall sense of satisfaction and happiness, as well as increase our chances of achieving success.

Overcoming Fear and Building Confidence: Risk-taking requires courage and a willingness to face uncertainty. By taking risks and pushing ourselves beyond our perceived limits, we can develop greater self-confidence and overcome fears that may be holding us back. This increased confidence can help us achieve success in many areas of our lives, from pursuing new career opportunities to building stronger personal relationships.

Identifying and Seizing Opportunities: Taking risks can open up new opportunities that we may not have otherwise considered.

By being willing to take a chance, we may discover a new career path, business opportunity, or personal passion that can lead to greater success and happiness.

Learning from Failure: Taking risks also means that we may experience failure or setbacks along the way. However, these experiences can provide valuable learning opportunities that can help us achieve greater success in the future. By learning from our mistakes, we can develop resilience, adaptability, and a willingness to take calculated risks that can lead to greater happiness and success.

Challenging the Status Quo: Taking risks often involves challenging the status quo or conventional wisdom. By questioning the norm and pursuing new and innovative ideas, we can create positive change in our lives and in the world around us. This can lead to greater fulfillment and a sense of purpose, as well as contribute to overall happiness and success.

Therefore, taking risks can have a powerful impact on achieving success and happiness. By being willing to step outside our comfort zones, challenge ourselves, and pursue new opportunities, we can develop the skills, confidence, and resilience necessary for long-term success and happiness.

How Taking Risk Lead to Unique Experiences and Opportunities

Taking risks can often lead to unique experiences and opportunities that we may not have otherwise encountered. Here are some ways in which taking risks can open up new and exciting opportunities:

Expanding Your Comfort Zone: When we take risks, we challenge ourselves to step outside our comfort zones and try something new. This can lead to unique experiences, such as traveling to a new destination, trying a new hobby, or exploring a new career path. By expanding our comfort zone, we can open up new opportunities for personal and professional growth.

Building New Relationships: Taking risks can also help us build new relationships with people who share similar interests or goals. By pursuing new opportunities, we may meet new people who can provide valuable insights, connections, and support that can lead to exciting new opportunities.

Discovering New Passions: When we take risks, we may discover new passions or interests that we may not have otherwise considered. For example, trying a new sport or activity may lead to a newfound love for outdoor adventure, while pursuing a new career path may lead to a passion for entrepreneurship or creative work.

Creating Innovative Solutions: Taking risks often involves challenging the status quo and pursuing new and innovative ideas. By pushing ourselves to think outside the box, we may discover unique solutions to problems or opportunities that can lead to exciting new ventures or projects.

Facing New Challenges: Taking risks can also involve facing new challenges and overcoming obstacles. While this can be intimidating, it can also be an opportunity to develop new skills, build resilience, and achieve personal growth. By embracing challenges and pushing ourselves to succeed, we can open up new opportunities and experiences that can lead to greater success and fulfillment.

Taking risks can lead to unique experiences and opportunities that can enhance our personal and professional lives. By being willing to step outside our comfort zones and pursue new and exciting opportunities, we can create a life full of adventure, growth, and fulfillment.

The Psychology of Risk-Taking

The psychology of risk-taking refers to the study of the mental and emotional processes that drive individuals to take risks in their lives. It involves understanding the underlying motivations, emotions, and cognitive processes that influence an individual's decision-making when faced with risk.

One of the key factors in the psychology of risk-taking is the role of emotions. Emotions such as fear, excitement, and anticipation can all play a significant role in an individual's willingness to take risks. For example, the fear of missing out or the excitement of a potential reward may lead individuals to take risks that they might not otherwise consider.

Another important factor in the psychology of risk-taking is cognitive biases. These are patterns of thinking that can lead individuals to make decisions that are not based on objective analysis of the situation. For example, individuals may be more likely to take risks if they have previously experienced success, even if the current situation is different.

Personality traits can also play a significant role in the psychology of risk-taking. Individuals who are high in sensation seeking, for example, may be more likely to take risks in order to seek out novel and stimulating experiences. In contrast, individuals who are high in conscientiousness may be more cautious and risk-averse.

Cultural and social factors can also influence an individual's willingness to take risks. For example, cultural attitudes towards risk-taking can differ widely between different societies, and social pressures can also play a role in shaping an individual's risk-taking behavior.

The psychology of risk-taking is a complex and multifaceted area of study that draws on a wide range of disciplines, including psychology, neuroscience, economics, and sociology. Understanding the psychology of risk-taking can be useful in a variety of contexts, from personal decision-making to risk management in organizations.

The Role of The Brain in Risk-Taking Behavior

The brain plays a critical role in risk-taking behavior, as it is responsible for processing information and making decisions based on that information. Here are some ways in which the brain influences risk-taking behavior:

Reward and Pleasure Centers: When we take risks, our brains release neurotransmitters such as dopamine, which are associated with reward and pleasure. This can create a sense of excitement and motivation to pursue risky behaviors, such as gambling or extreme sports.

Fear and Anxiety Centers: At the same time, the brain also has fear and anxiety centers that can signal potential danger or risk. These centers may become activated when we face uncertain or unfamiliar situations, causing us to feel fear or anxiety that can influence our decision-making.

Rational Decision-Making: In addition to emotional responses, the brain also plays a role in rational decision-making. The prefrontal cortex is responsible for weighing the pros and cons of a decision and considering potential outcomes. This area of the brain can help us make calculated risks that have the potential for positive outcomes.

Experience and Memory: The brain also uses past experiences and memories to inform decision-making. If we have had positive experiences with risky behavior in the past, we may be more likely to engage in that behavior again. Similarly, if we have had negative experiences, we may be more cautious or avoidant of that behavior in the future.

Genetics and Personality: Finally, genetics and personality can also influence risk-taking behavior. Some individuals may have a genetic predisposition to seeking out novel or risky experiences, while others may be more risk-averse due to personality traits such as conscientiousness or neuroticism.

The brain plays a complex role in risk-taking behavior, as it involves a combination of emotional responses, rational decision-making, past experiences, and genetics/personality. By understanding these factors, we can better understand why we may be drawn to certain risky behaviors and how we can make informed decisions about our behavior.

The effects of personality traits, such as openness to experience and conscientiousness, on risk-taking behaviour

Personality traits can have a significant impact on risk-taking behavior. Here are some ways in which traits such as openness to experience and conscientiousness can influence risk-taking:

- Openness to Experience: Openness to experience is a personality trait characterized by a willingness to try new things, Accept new ideas, and seek out novelty. Individuals who score high in openness to experience may be more likely to engage in risky behaviors, such as trying new drugs, pursuing unconventional careers, or engaging in extreme sports.

- Conscientiousness: Conscientiousness is a personality trait characterized by organization, self-discipline, and responsibility.

Individuals who score high in consciousness may be less likely to engage in risky behaviors, as they are more focused on achieving their goals and following rules and norms.

- Moderating Factors: While openness to experience and conscientiousness can have a significant impact on risk-taking behavior, it is important to note that other factors can also play a role. For example, individuals who score high in openness to experience may be less likely to take risks if they have strong social support networks that discourage risky behavior. Similarly, individuals who score high in conscientiousness may be more likely to take risks if they are in high-stress situations or feel pressured to succeed.

- Gender Differences: Studies have also shown that gender can influence the relationship between personality traits and risk-taking behavior. For example, men may be more likely to engage in risky behaviors, regardless of their personality traits, while women may be more influenced by their personality traits in their decision-making.

- Developmental Changes: Finally, it is important to note that personality traits and risk-taking behavior can change over time. For example, individuals may become more risk-averse as they age, or may become more willing to take risks as they gain experience and confidence.

Personality traits such as openness to experience and conscientiousness can have a significant impact on risk-taking behavior. By understanding how these traits influence our decision-making, we can make more informed choices about our behavior and take steps to mitigate potential risks.

Influence of past experiences and upbringing on risk-taking behaviour

Past experiences and upbringing can have a significant influence on risk-taking behavior. Here are some ways in which these factors can affect our decision-making:

Learned Behavior: One way in which past experiences and upbringing can influence risk-taking behavior is through learned behavior. For example, if we grew up in an environment where risk-taking behavior was encouraged or rewarded, we may be more likely to engage in such behavior ourselves. Similarly, if we have had positive experiences with risky behavior in the past, we may be more likely to continue that behavior in the future.

Fear and Trauma: On the other hand, past experiences can also lead to fear and trauma that can impact our willingness to take risks. For example, if we have had negative experiences with risky behavior, such as a traumatic injury, we may be more cautious or avoidant of similar behavior in the future.

Social Norms: Upbringing and past experiences can also influence our perception of social norms and expectations around risk-taking behavior. For example, if we were raised in a culture that values risk-taking and innovation, we may be more likely to engage in risky behavior to meet those expectations. Conversely, if we were raised in a culture that values caution and stability, we may be more risk-averse.

Personal Values: Past experiences and upbringing can also shape our personal values, which can influence our decision-making around risk-taking behavior. For example, if we were raised with a strong sense of responsibility and duty, we may be less likely to engage in behavior that could put ourselves or others at risk.

Overcoming Negative Influences: While past experiences and upbringing can have a significant impact on risk-taking behavior, it is important to note that we can also take steps to overcome negative influences. For example, by seeking out positive role models or seeking therapy to address trauma or anxiety, we can work to develop a more balanced and informed approach to risk-taking.

Past experiences and upbringing can have a significant influence on risk-taking behavior. By understanding how these factors shape our decision-making, we can work to develop a more conscious and intentional approach to risk-taking.

Types of Risks

Mainly three types of risk are prevalent - Financial, Emotional, Professional, and Personal.

Financial Risk

In the early 2000s, Elon Musk co-founded PayPal, a company that revolutionized online payments. However, instead of playing it safe and enjoying the profits from PayPal, Musk decided to take a risk and invest in his dream of colonizing Mars.

He founded SpaceX in 2002, with the goal of reducing the cost of space exploration and eventually making life multi-planetary. The company faced many challenges along the way, including multiple failed launches and rocket explosions. But Musk persisted, and eventually achieved many milestones, including the first privately-funded spacecraft to reach orbit, and the first privately-funded spacecraft to dock with the International Space Station.

While Musk's investment in SpaceX was risky, it ultimately paid off. The company now has a market valuation of over $74 billion and has made major contributions to space exploration. Musk's story is a prime example of how taking calculated financial risks can lead to great success.

Financial risk is the risk of losing money or assets due to factors such as market fluctuations, fraud, or default. Financial risk refers to the possibility of financial loss or failure due to factors such as market fluctuations, currency exchange rates, and credit or liquidity risks. Here are some examples of financial risk:

Market Risk: Market risk refers to the possibility of loss due to changes in market conditions, such as changes in interest rates, stock prices, or commodity prices. For example, if an investor has a portfolio heavily invested in stocks, they may face significant financial losses if the stock market experiences a downturn.

Credit Risk: Credit risk refers to the possibility of loss due to the failure of a borrower to repay a loan or debt. For example, if a bank lends money to a borrower who later defaults on their payments, the bank may face financial losses.

Liquidity Risk: Liquidity risk refers to the possibility of loss due to the inability to sell an asset quickly and at a fair price. For example, if an investor holds a large position in a relatively illiquid stock, they may face difficulty selling that stock quickly if market conditions change.

Foreign Exchange Risk: Foreign exchange risk refers to the possibility of loss due to changes in currency exchange rates. For example, if a company based in the United States sells products to customers in Europe, they may face financial losses if the

Euro depreciates significantly against the U.S. dollar.

Interest Rate Risk: Interest rate risk refers to the possibility of loss due to changes in interest rates. For example, if an investor holds bonds with fixed interest rates and interest rates rise, the market value of those bonds may decline.

Inflation Risk: Inflation risk refers to the possibility of loss due to inflation reducing the purchasing power of money. For example, if an investor holds cash in a low-interest savings account, the value of that cash may be eroded over time due to inflation.

The financial risk can take many different forms, and can arise from a variety of factors. By understanding these risks, individuals and organizations can take steps to manage and mitigate them, and make more informed financial decisions.

Strategic Risk

One real-life example of strategic risk is Netflix's decision to shift its focus from renting DVDs to online streaming. In 2011, Netflix faced significant backlash when it announced a price increase for its DVD and streaming plans, which resulted in a large number of customer cancellations. In response, Netflix shifted its focus solely to online streaming and invested heavily in creating original content. This decision was a strategic risk because it required a significant investment of time and money, and there was no guarantee that it would pay off. However, the move ultimately paid off, as Netflix became the dominant player in the online streaming market, with a market capitalization of over $250 billion as of 2021. This example highlights the importance of taking strategic risks in order to stay competitive and adapt to changing market conditions.

Strategic risk is the risk of making decisions that negatively impact an organization's long-term goals or reputation. Examples of strategic risk include entering a new market without proper research or investing in a project that ultimately fails.

Social Risk

Rosa Parks was an African American woman who, in 1955, refused to give up her seat on a Montgomery, Alabama bus to a white person, as was required by local segregation laws. This act of defiance sparked the Montgomery Bus Boycott, which was a pivotal moment in the civil rights movement.

Parks took a significant social risk by refusing to comply with the discriminatory laws of the time. She faced arrest and potential violence, as well as being ostracized by her community. However, by taking this risk, she became a symbol of resistance to segregation and helped to bring about lasting change. Her actions and the resulting boycott ultimately led to a Supreme Court ruling that declared segregation on public buses to be unconstitutional. Parks' social risk-taking serves as a powerful example of how individuals can use their actions to challenge injustice and effect change.

Social risk refers to the risk of loss resulting from negative social or political factors, such as public protests, boycotts, and government regulation.

Social risk refers to the possibility of social rejection, disapproval, or ostracism that can arise from taking certain actions or expressing certain beliefs. Here are some examples of social risks:

Challenging social norms: Challenging social norms, such as gender roles or cultural traditions, can be a social risk as it can lead to disapproval or rejection from others who adhere to those norms. For example, advocating for gender equality or expressing support for a marginalized group can be socially risky in certain contexts.

Expressing unpopular opinions: Expressing an opinion that goes against the prevailing views of a group or community can be a social risk, as it can lead to criticism or ostracism from others. For example, expressing support for a political candidate or a controversial social issue can be socially risky.

Coming out: Coming out as LGBTQ+ or disclosing a marginalized identity can be a social risk, as it can lead to rejection or discrimination from others who hold negative attitudes towards those identities.

Standing up to bullying or harassment: Standing up to bullying or harassment can be a social risk, as it can lead to retaliation or further mistreatment from the bully or their supporters. For example, speaking out against workplace harassment or confronting a cyberbully can be socially risky.

Starting a new social group or activity: Starting a new social group or activity, such as a hobby group or a social club, can be a social risk as it involves putting oneself out there and potentially facing rejection or disinterest from others.

Social risks involve the possibility of social rejection or disapproval that can arise from taking certain actions or expressing certain beliefs. However, taking social risks can also lead to personal growth, social change, and the formation of meaningful connections with others who share similar values and beliefs.

Emotional risk

One real life story of emotional risk involves the American singer and actress, Lady Gaga. In the early days of her career, Lady Gaga faced a lot of criticism and rejection from record labels and producers who felt that her music and image were too unconventional and risky. However, Lady Gaga remained committed to her vision and took emotional risks by constantly pushing boundaries and challenging the status quo.

In an interview with Oprah Winfrey, Lady Gaga revealed that she struggled with depression and anxiety as a result of the pressures of fame and the emotional toll of constantly being judged and criticized. However, she used these experiences to fuel her music and connect with her fans on a deeper level. She also became a vocal advocate for mental health awareness and encouraged her fans to Accept their differences and find strength in vulnerability.

Through her willingness to take emotional risks and be true to herself, Lady Gaga has become one of the most successful and influential musicians of her generation, inspiring millions of fans around the world to Accept their own unique identities and overcome their own emotional challenges.

Emotional risk refers to the possibility of emotional or psychological harm that can arise from taking certain actions or decisions. Here are some examples of emotional risks:

Vulnerability: Being vulnerable and opening up to others can be an emotional risk, as it can make us feel exposed and potentially rejected or hurt. For example, telling a loved one about your deepest fears or sharing a personal struggle with a friend can be emotionally risky.

Rejection: Taking a chance and putting yourself out there, whether it be in a personal or professional context, can lead to rejection. For example, applying for a job or asking someone on a date both involve the risk of rejection, which can be emotionally challenging.

Speaking up: Speaking up for what you believe in or challenging the status quo can be an emotional risk, as it can lead to conflict or pushback from others. For example, speaking up about a workplace issue or voicing a dissenting opinion in a group discussion can be emotionally risky.

Change: Making changes in your life, whether it be a career change, a move to a new city, or starting a new relationship, can be emotionally risky. These changes can be uncertain and can bring up feelings of fear or anxiety.

Trusting others: Trusting others, whether it be a friend, family member, or romantic partner, can be emotionally risky. Trusting someone means opening yourself up to the possibility of betrayal or disappointment.

In nutshell, emotional risks involve putting oneself in a vulnerable position, which can lead to emotional or psychological harm. However, taking emotional risks can also lead to personal growth and fulfilling experiences, and can help individuals build resilience and develop coping skills.

Health and Safety Risk:

One example of a health and safety risk is the story of Aron Ralston, a hiker who became trapped in a narrow canyon in Utah in 2003. While climbing, a boulder dislodged and trapped his right hand against the canyon wall. He was stuck there for five days without food or water, until he eventually decided to amputate his own arm in order to free himself and seek help.

Ralston's story highlights the physical and emotional risks associated with outdoor activities and adventure sports. His lack of preparation and safety precautions put him in a dangerous situation, and his decision to take a drastic step to save himself illustrates the extreme measures that people may take in order to manage health and safety risks.

Health and safety risk refers to the risk of loss resulting from accidents or incidents that harm employees, customers, or the public. This can include risks related to workplace safety, food safety, and product safety.

Health and safety risks refer to the possibility of harm or injury to oneself or others in the workplace, home, or other environments. Here are some examples of health and safety risks:

Physical hazards: Physical hazards refer to the potential for physical harm or injury, such as slips and falls, cuts, burns, or exposure to harmful substances. For example, working with machinery without proper safety precautions, handling chemicals without protective gear, or walking on a slippery surface can be physical hazards.

Ergonomic hazards: Ergonomic hazards refer to the potential for harm or injury related to the design of workstations or equipment. For example, repetitive motions, awkward postures, and heavy lifting can cause musculoskeletal disorders.

Biological hazards: Biological hazards refer to the potential for harm or injury related to exposure to infectious agents, such as viruses, bacteria, or fungi. For example, exposure to bloodborne pathogens in a healthcare setting or foodborne illness from contaminated food can be biological hazards.

Environmental hazards: Environmental hazards refer to the potential for harm or injury related to exposure to natural or man-made hazards in the environment, such as extreme weather conditions, radiation, or pollution. For example, exposure to air pollution in a high-traffic area or working in extreme temperatures can be environmental hazards.

Psychosocial hazards: Psychosocial hazards refer to the potential for harm or injury related to work-related stress, harassment, or violence. For example, workplace bullying or exposure to traumatic events in a high-stress job can be psychosocial hazards.

Health and safety risks refer to the potential for harm or injury in the workplace, home, or other environments. Taking precautions and following safety guidelines can help mitigate these risks and prevent accidents or injuries.

Reputational Risk:

One example of a reputational risk is the case of BP's Deepwater Horizon oil spill in 2010. BP faced not only environmental and financial risks but also a major reputational risk. The oil spill caused extensive damage to the environment, harming wildlife and disrupting the lives of thousands of people living in the affected areas.

BP's response to the spill was widely criticized, and the company faced public outrage and scrutiny from government agencies, investors, and other stakeholders. The spill caused significant damage to BP's reputation, and the company had to undertake a massive public relations effort to restore its image.

BP's CEO at the time, Tony Hayward, famously stated that he wanted his life back while the oil spill continued to rage on. His comment was seen as insensitive and tone-deaf, further damaging the company's reputation. In the aftermath of the spill, BP faced multiple lawsuits and regulatory fines, which took a toll on its financial performance.

The Deepwater Horizon oil spill serves as a cautionary tale about the importance of managing reputational risk. Companies need to be prepared to deal with crises and communicate effectively with stakeholders to avoid damaging their reputation.

Volkswagen Emissions Scandal: In 2015, Volkswagen (VW) admitted to installing software in their diesel cars to cheat on emissions tests. This scandal led to a loss of trust in the company and a decline in sales. VW was forced to pay billions of dollars in settlements and fines and their reputation was severely damaged.

Wells Fargo Fake Accounts Scandal: In 2016, it was discovered that Wells Fargo employees had opened millions of fake accounts without customers' knowledge in order to meet sales quotas. This scandal led to a loss of trust in the bank and a decline in its stock price. Wells Fargo was fined billions of dollars and its CEO resigned.

United Airlines Passenger Removal Incident: In 2017, a United Airlines passenger was violently removed from a flight after refusing to give up his seat. The incident was captured on video and went viral, leading to a public outcry and a boycott of the airline. United Airlines' stock price dropped and the company's reputation was damaged.

Nestle Baby Formula Controversy: In the 1970s, Nestle was accused of promoting its baby formula in developing countries, where it was not safe to use due to unsanitary water and lack of knowledge on how to prepare it properly. This led to a boycott of Nestle products and a loss of trust in the company. Nestle eventually changed its marketing practices and introduced new safety measures, but the controversy damaged its reputation for years.

Reputational risk is the risk of damage to an organization's reputation or brand value due to factors such as negative publicity, product recalls, or ethical violations.

Reputation risk refers to the possibility of negative public perception or damage to one's reputation due to certain actions, decisions, or events. Here are some examples of reputation risks:

Ethical violations: Ethical violations, such as fraud, corruption, or data breaches, can damage an organization's reputation and erode public trust. For example, a financial institution caught in a scandal involving unethical practices can lead to a loss of customers and damage to the company's reputation.

Product recalls: Product recalls due to safety concerns or defects can damage a company's reputation, as it suggests that the company did not take sufficient precautions to ensure product quality and safety. For example, a car company that recalls a large number of vehicles due to safety issues can damage its reputation and lead to a loss of customers.

Negative media coverage: Negative media coverage, such as critical news articles or social media posts, can damage an individual's or organization's reputation. For example, a politician caught in a scandal or a celebrity caught engaging in inappropriate behavior can face negative media coverage that damages their reputation.

Stakeholder dissatisfaction: Stakeholder dissatisfaction, such as employee grievances or customer complaints, can damage an organization's reputation. For example, a restaurant that receives negative reviews due to poor customer service or food quality can damage its reputation and lead to a loss of customers.

Environmental impact: Environmental impact, such as pollution or environmental damage, can damage an organization's reputation, especially if the organization is perceived as not taking sufficient steps to mitigate environmental harm. For example, an oil company that is involved in an oil spill can face damage to its reputation and public scrutiny.

Reputation risk refers to the possibility of negative public perception or damage to one's reputation due to certain actions, decisions, or events. Mitigating reputation risk involves taking steps to ensure ethical conduct, product quality, customer satisfaction, and environmental responsibility.

Legal Risk:

One real-life example of legal risk can be seen in the case of Enron, a former energy and commodities company that filed for bankruptcy in 2001. Enron's top executives were found guilty of financial fraud and other criminal charges, resulting in the company being dissolved and many of its former employees losing their jobs and retirement savings. This legal risk also had a significant impact on the reputation of the accounting firm Arthur Andersen, which was found guilty of obstruction of justice for its role in the scandal and subsequently went out of business.

Another example of legal risk can be seen in the tobacco industry. Many tobacco companies have faced lawsuits for selling products that were known to cause cancer and other health problems. These lawsuits have resulted in large fines and settlements, as well as negative publicity that has damaged the reputation of the companies involved.

Compliance risk is the risk of legal or regulatory penalties due to failure to comply with laws and regulations. Examples of compliance risk include violations of environmental regulations or labor laws.

Legal risk refers to the possibility of financial or legal consequences due to non-compliance with laws, regulations, or contractual obligations. Here are some examples of legal risks:

Contractual breaches: A breach of contract occurs when one party fails to fulfill the terms of a contract. This can lead to legal action by the other party, which can result in financial damages or other legal consequences.

Intellectual property infringement: Intellectual property infringement occurs when a company uses someone else's patented or copyrighted material without permission. This can result in legal action by the owner of the intellectual property, which can lead to fines or other legal consequences.

Regulatory compliance violations: Regulatory compliance violations occur when a company fails to comply with laws or regulations that govern its industry. This can result in legal action by regulatory agencies, which can lead to fines or other legal consequences.

Employee disputes: Employee disputes can lead to legal action by employees, which can result in financial damages or other legal consequences. For example, an employee who is wrongfully terminated or discriminated against can file a lawsuit against the employer.

Product liability: Product liability occurs when a company's product causes harm or injury to a consumer. This can result in legal action by the consumer, which can lead to financial damages or other legal consequences.

Therefore, legal risk refers to the possibility of financial or legal consequences due to non-compliance with laws, regulations, or contractual obligations. Mitigating legal risk involves ensuring compliance with applicable laws and regulations, carefully reviewing contracts and agreements, and maintaining appropriate insurance coverage.

Relationship Between Different Types of Risks

Different types of risks are often interconnected, and one type of risk can have an impact on another. Here are some examples of how different types of risks can impact each other:

Financial risk and reputation risk: A company that takes on excessive financial risk may experience negative financial outcomes, which can damage its reputation. For example, a company that takes on too much debt may struggle to make loan payments, which can damage its reputation and make it difficult to attract investors.

Health and safety risk and legal risk: A company that fails to ensure the health and safety of its employees may be at risk of facing legal action by regulatory agencies or employees. For example, if a company fails to provide appropriate safety equipment to its employees, it may be subject to fines or other legal consequences.

Social risk and reputation risk: A company that engages in practices that are perceived as socially irresponsible may face negative public perception, which can damage its reputation. For example, a company that is found to use child labor or engage in discriminatory practices may face negative media coverage, which can damage its reputation and lead to a loss of customers.

Emotional risk and health and safety risk: An individual who takes on excessive emotional risk, such as by ignoring stress or burnout, may experience negative health outcomes, such as mental health issues or physical illness. For example, an employee who works long hours without taking breaks or addressing workplace stress may be at risk of developing health problems.

Mitigating risk involves identifying potential risks and taking appropriate steps to manage them, including implementing risk management strategies and maintaining appropriate insurance coverage.

Prioritizing Risk

In 2005, Hurricane Katrina hit the Gulf Coast of the United States and caused widespread damage and loss of life. The disaster highlighted the importance of prioritizing risks and investing in preventative measures. Experts had long warned that New Orleans was at risk of flooding due to its location below sea level, but funding for infrastructure improvements was not prioritized. As a result, when Katrina hit, the city's levee system failed, resulting in catastrophic flooding.

Identifying and prioritizing different types of risks is important for individuals and organizations to effectively manage their risks. Here are some steps to identify and prioritize risks based on individual circumstances:

Conduct a risk assessment: A risk assessment involves identifying potential risks and assessing the likelihood and potential impact of each risk. This can be done through a formal process that includes gathering data, analyzing potential scenarios, and assessing the likelihood of each risk.

Categorize risks: Once potential risks have been identified, categorize them into different types of risks, such as financial, legal, or health and safety risks. This can help in prioritizing risks based on their potential impact on your life or organization.

Prioritize risks: Prioritize risks based on their potential impact and likelihood. Some risks may have a high impact but a low likelihood of occurring, while others may have a low impact but a high likelihood of occurring. Consider the consequences of each risk and the resources available to manage them.

Develop risk management strategies: Once risks have been identified and prioritized, develop risk management strategies to mitigate the impact of the risks. This may include implementing risk management policies, developing contingency plans, or purchasing insurance.

Review and update the risk assessment regularly: Risks and circumstances can change over time, so it's important to review and update the risk assessment regularly to ensure that risks are properly identified and managed.

Identifying and prioritizing different types of risks based on individual circumstances involves conducting a risk assessment, categorizing risks, prioritizing risks, developing risk management strategies, and reviewing and updating the risk assessment regularly. This process can help individuals and organizations effectively manage their risks and minimize their impact.

Calculated Risks

One example of a calculated risk is the story of Sara Blakely, the founder of Spanx. In the late 1990s, Blakely came up with the idea for women's shapewear that was comfortable, seamless, and could be worn under white pants. She had no experience in the fashion industry but believed in her product and decided to invest her entire life savings of $5,000 to develop a prototype. She then pitched her product to various manufacturers and potential investors, receiving multiple rejections.

However, Blakely persisted and eventually secured a deal with a hosiery manufacturer. She launched her product in high-end department stores and quickly gained a following. Today, Spanx is a highly successful and profitable company with over $400 million in annual revenue.

Blakely took a calculated risk by investing her life savings in her idea and pursuing it despite facing rejection. She weighed the potential consequences of failure against the opportunity for success and ultimately made the decision to take the risk. Her determination and willingness to take calculated risks ultimately led to her success.

The founders of McDonald's, Richard and Maurice McDonald, took a calculated risk when they decided to franchise their successful fast-food restaurant in the 1950s. They carefully selected franchisees and created a system that ensured consistency and quality across all locations. This risk paid off, and McDonald's is now one of the largest and most successful fast-food chains in the world.

Calculated risks refer to the process of making a decision to take a risk after carefully analyzing the potential opportunity and consequence. This means that instead of taking a blind leap of faith, you weigh the potential benefits against the potential risks and make a more informed decision.

Here are some steps to take when balancing opportunity and consequence to take calculated risks:

Define the opportunity: Start by clearly defining the opportunity you are considering. This may be a new business venture, a job opportunity, or an investment.

Assess the potential benefits: Analyze the potential benefits of taking the risk. This may include financial gain, personal growth, or career advancement.

Identify the potential consequences: Identify the potential consequences of taking the risk. This may include financial loss, personal setbacks, or damage to your reputation.

Determine the likelihood of success: Assess the likelihood of success based on your skills, resources, and experience.

Determine the level of risk tolerance: Evaluate your level of risk tolerance and determine how much risk you are willing to take.

Weigh the potential benefits against the potential consequences: Consider the potential benefits and consequences of taking the risk, and weigh them against each other.

Make an informed decision: Based on the analysis, make an informed decision on whether to take the risk or not. If you decide to take the risk, develop a plan to manage and mitigate the potential consequences.

Taking calculated risks involves carefully analyzing the potential benefits and consequences of a decision before making a well-informed decision. By balancing opportunity and consequence, individuals can make more informed decisions and minimize the potential negative impact of taking risks.

How to evaluate the potential outcomes of a risk

To evaluate the potential outcomes of a risk, here are some steps you can take:

Identify the risk: First, identify the risk you are evaluating. This may be a business decision, an investment, or a personal decision.

Consider the potential outcomes: Consider the potential outcomes of taking the risk. This includes both positive and negative outcomes.

Determine the likelihood of each outcome: Consider the likelihood of each outcome occurring. This may require research and data analysis.

Assess the impact of each outcome: Assess the impact of each outcome on your goals, resources, and well-being.

Evaluate the risk-reward ratio: Evaluate the risk-reward ratio of each outcome. This means weighing the potential rewards against the potential risks and determining if the potential rewards are worth the potential risks.

Develop a risk management plan: Develop a risk management plan to mitigate the potential negative impact of the risk. This may include implementing risk control measures or developing contingency plans.

Monitor and evaluate the outcomes: Monitor and evaluate the outcomes of the risk. This will help you determine if the potential outcomes were accurately evaluated and if the risk management plan was effective.

In short, evaluating the potential outcomes of a risk involves considering the potential outcomes, determining the likelihood and impact of each outcome, evaluating the risk-reward ratio, developing a risk management plan, and monitoring and evaluating the outcomes. By evaluating the potential outcomes, individuals can make more informed decisions and mitigate the potential negative impact of taking risks.

How to Determine The Probability of Success and Failure

To determine the probability of success and failure, you can follow these steps:

Identify the potential outcomes: Start by identifying the potential outcomes of the decision or action you are considering. For example, if you are considering starting a new business venture, the potential outcomes could be success or failure.

Analyze the factors influencing the outcomes: Identify the factors that could influence the outcome. For example, if you are starting a new business, factors such as market demand, competition, and your own skills and resources could influence the outcome.

Assign a probability to each factor: Assign a probability to each factor based on your assessment of its likelihood. For example, if you determine that market demand for your product is high, you might assign a higher probability of success.

Multiply the probabilities: Multiply the probabilities of each factor to determine the overall probability of success or failure. For example, if you assign a 70% probability to high market demand, and a 60% probability to your own skills and resources, the overall probability of success would be 42% (0.7 x 0.6 = 0.42).

Evaluate the risk-reward ratio: Evaluate the risk-reward ratio by weighing the potential rewards against the potential risks. If the probability of success is high and the potential rewards are substantial, the risk-reward ratio may be favorable.

Develop a risk management plan: Develop a risk management plan to mitigate the potential negative impact of failure. This may include developing contingency plans or implementing risk control measures.

By following these steps, you can more accurately determine the probability of success and failure of a decision or action, and make a more informed decision about whether or not to take the risk.

How to Make Informed Decisions Based on Careful Analysis and Preparation

To make informed decisions based on careful analysis and preparation, follow these steps:

Define the problem or decision: Start by defining the problem or decision you need to make. Be clear about what you want to achieve and why it matters.

Gather information: Gather as much relevant information as possible about the problem or decision. This could include data, research, and expert opinions. Be sure to gather information from multiple sources to ensure you have a comprehensive understanding.

Analyze the information: Analyze the information you have gathered and identify patterns and trends. This will help you to identify potential solutions and weigh the pros and cons of each.

Consider alternatives: Consider alternatives to the solution you have identified. Weigh the advantages and disadvantages of each alternative.

Determine potential outcomes: Determine the potential outcomes of each alternative. Consider both the short-term and long-term consequences of each.

Evaluate the risks: Evaluate the risks associated with each alternative. Consider the potential impact on your goals, resources, and well-being.

Make a decision: Based on your analysis and evaluation, make a decision. Choose the alternative that has the greatest potential for success and the lowest risk.

Develop an action plan: Develop an action plan to implement your decision. Identify the steps you need to take, the resources you need, and the timeline for completion.

Monitor and evaluate: Monitor and evaluate the progress of your decision. This will help you to make adjustments if necessary and ensure that you are on track to achieve your goals.

By following these steps, you can make informed decisions based on careful analysis and preparation. This will help you to achieve your goals with the least amount of risk and the greatest potential for success.

Understanding the Role of Fear in Risk-taking

One real-life example of how fear can be an obstacle to taking risks is the story of J.K. Rowling, the author of the Harry Potter series. Before the publication of the first Harry Potter book, Rowling faced numerous rejections from publishers who were skeptical that a children's book about wizards would sell. Despite this, Rowling continued to write and submit her manuscript, showing persistence in the face of rejection.

However, even after finding a publisher, Rowling continued to experience fear and self-doubt. She was afraid of how her book would be received by the public and worried that she was not a good enough writer. These fears could have prevented her from promoting her book and pursuing opportunities to expand the Harry Potter franchise. Instead, she faced her fears and went on a book tour, speaking to fans and promoting her work. This led to the enormous success of the series and the creation of a multi-billion dollar franchise. Rowling's example shows that even when fear is present, it is possible to overcome it and take risks that can lead to great rewards.

Fear plays a crucial role in risk-taking because it is a natural human response to perceived danger. Fear is an instinctive response to potential threats or harm, and it is hard-wired into our brains as a survival mechanism. When faced with a risky situation, fear can trigger the fight-or-flight response, which prepares the body to respond to danger.

However, fear can also hold us back from taking risks and trying new things. The fear of failure, rejection, or uncertainty can be paralyzing, preventing us from pursuing opportunities that could lead to growth and success.

To understand the role of fear in risk-taking, it's important to recognize that fear is not necessarily a bad thing. It can be a useful tool to help us assess risks and make informed decisions. However, when fear becomes excessive or irrational, it can prevent us from taking necessary risks and pursuing our goals.

To overcome fear and take calculated risks, it's important to recognize the difference between real and perceived threats. Often, our fears are based on assumptions and beliefs that are not based in reality. By challenging these beliefs and examining the evidence, we can gain a more accurate understanding of the risks involved and make informed decisions.

It's also helpful to reframe our thinking around risk-taking. Instead of focusing on the potential negative outcomes, we can focus on the potential rewards and benefits. By reframing our thinking in this way, we can build confidence and resilience, and become more comfortable with taking risks.

In summary, fear plays a critical role in risk-taking, but it's important to recognize that fear is not necessarily a bad thing. By understanding the role of fear in risk-taking, challenging our assumptions and beliefs, and reframing our thinking, we can overcome fear and take calculated risks to achieve our goals.

Managing anxiety is an essential part of being able to take calculated risks. Anxiety can be a significant barrier to risk-taking, as it can prevent individuals from feeling confident and making clear decisions. Here are some techniques for managing anxiety:

Mindfulness: Mindfulness is a technique that involves paying attention to the present moment without judgment. Practicing mindfulness can help individuals stay calm and focused, reducing feelings of anxiety.

Deep Breathing: Deep breathing is a technique that can help individuals slow down their heart rate and calm their nervous system. Taking deep breaths can help individuals feel more centered and relaxed.

Progressive Muscle Relaxation: Progressive muscle relaxation is a technique that involves tensing and relaxing specific muscle groups in the body. This technique can help individuals release tension and feel more relaxed.

Cognitive Behavioral Therapy: Cognitive-behavioral therapy (CBT) is a type of therapy that can help individuals manage anxiety by changing their thoughts and behaviors. CBT can help individuals identify negative thought patterns and replace them with more positive ones.

Exercise: Regular exercise can help individuals reduce feelings of anxiety and stress. Exercise can also increase the body's production of endorphins, which are natural mood-boosters.

Healthy Lifestyle: Maintaining a healthy lifestyle can also help individuals manage anxiety. This includes getting enough sleep, eating a healthy diet, and avoiding substances that can increase anxiety, such as caffeine and alcohol.

Support Network: Having a support network of friends, family, or a therapist can also be helpful in managing anxiety. Having someone to talk to can help individuals feel less alone and provide perspective on their concerns.

Managing anxiety is essential to taking calculated risks. Techniques such as mindfulness, deep breathing, progressive muscle relaxation, cognitive-behavioral therapy, exercise, healthy lifestyle, and support networks can all be helpful in managing anxiety.

How to Build Resilience and Develop a Growth Mindset

Building resilience and developing a growth mindset are important aspects of being able to take risks and manage the outcomes of those risks. Here are some tips for building resilience and developing a growth mindset:

Accept Challenges: Challenges are an opportunity to learn and grow. Embracing challenges and viewing them as opportunities can help individuals build resilience and develop a growth mindset.

Focus on the Positive: Focusing on the positive aspects of a situation can help individuals build resilience and maintain a growth mindset. This involves reframing negative thoughts and finding the silver lining in difficult situations.

Practice Self-Care: Taking care of oneself is essential for building resilience and maintaining a growth mindset. This includes getting enough sleep, eating a healthy diet, exercising regularly, and taking time to relax and recharge.

Learn from Failure: Failure is a natural part of taking risks. Learning from failure and using it as an opportunity to grow and improve can help individuals build resilience and develop a growth mindset.

Practice Mindfulness: Mindfulness can help individuals stay focused on the present moment and reduce feelings of stress and anxiety. Practicing mindfulness can help individuals build resilience and develop a growth mindset.

Build a Support Network: Having a support network of friends, family, or colleagues can be helpful in building resilience and maintaining a growth mindset. Having people to turn to during difficult times can help individuals feel less alone and more supported.

Set Realistic Goals: Setting realistic goals can help individuals build resilience and maintain a growth mindset. Setting goals that are too lofty can lead to disappointment and feelings of failure, while setting achievable goals can help individuals build confidence and momentum.

Building resilience and developing a growth mindset are essential for taking risks and managing the outcomes of those risks. Embracing challenges, focusing on the positive, practicing self-care, learning from failure, practicing mindfulness, cultivating a support network, and setting realistic goals are all ways to build resilience and develop a growth mindset.

The Importance of Failure

One great story on learning from mistakes is that of Thomas Edison, the inventor of the electric light bulb. Edison was known for his persistence and his willingness to take risks. In his quest to invent the light bulb, Edison conducted thousands of experiments, many of which failed. He once said, "I have not failed. I've just found 10,000 ways that won't work."

Edison saw each failure as an opportunity to learn and improve his approach. He kept detailed records of his experiments and analyzed his results, using each failure to inform his next attempt. Finally, after years of trial and error, Edison was successful in creating a commercially viable electric light bulb.

Edison's story is a powerful example of the importance of learning from mistakes. By reframing his failures as opportunities to learn, Edison was able to stay focused and persistent in the face of adversity. He didn't let his mistakes discourage him, but instead used them as stepping stones on his path to success.

The Role Of Failure In The Process Of Taking Risks

Failure is an inevitable part of taking risks, and it plays a critical role in the process. Here are some ways that failure is important in the process of taking risks:

Failure is a Learning Opportunity: When we fail, we have an opportunity to learn from our mistakes and gain new insights that can help us improve our approach. We can reflect on what went wrong, identify areas for improvement, and adjust our approach for next time.

Failure Builds Resilience: When we experience failure, we learn how to cope with setbacks and bounce back from difficult situations. This resilience can help us to continue taking risks and pursuing our goals, even when faced with challenges.

Failure Encourages Innovation: When we take risks, we often try new things and experiment with different approaches. Failure can encourage us to think creatively and come up with innovative solutions to problems.

Failure Redefines Success: Failure can help us redefine what success means to us. We may realize that success is not always about achieving a specific outcome, but about the process of learning, growing, and pushing ourselves beyond our comfort zone.

Failure Provides Perspective: Failure can help us gain perspective and put things in context. It can remind us that taking risks is a part of life, and that setbacks and failures are not the end of the world. This can help us to be more resilient, optimistic, and adaptable in the face of future challenges.

Failure plays a critical role in the process of taking risks. It provides us with learning opportunities, builds resilience, encourages innovation, redefines success, and provides perspective. By embracing failure as a natural part of the risk-taking process, we can learn and grow from our experiences, and continue to pursue our goals with confidence and resilience.

Understanding the lessons that can be learned from failure

Failure can be a valuable teacher, and there are many lessons that can be learned from it. Here are some of the key lessons that can be learned from failure:

The Importance of Preparation: Failure can highlight the importance of preparation and planning. Often, failure is the result of insufficient preparation or a lack of attention to important details. By taking the time to prepare thoroughly, we can minimize the risk of failure and increase our chances of success.

The Value of Persistence: Failure can also teach us the value of persistence. When we experience setbacks or failures, it can be tempting to give up or become discouraged.

However, persistence can help us to continue pushing forward, even in the face of adversity.

The Need for Flexibility: Failure can also remind us of the need for flexibility and adaptability. Sometimes, our initial plans or approaches may not work out as intended, and we may need to adjust our strategies or try something new.

The Power of Positive Thinking: Failure can also highlight the importance of positive thinking. When we adopt a positive mindset, we are more likely to learn from our failures and use them as opportunities for growth and improvement.

The Benefits of Self-Reflection: Failure can also encourage self-reflection and introspection. By taking the time to reflect on our failures and mistakes, we can identify areas for improvement and develop new strategies for success.

Failure can be a powerful teacher, and there are many lessons that can be learned from it. By embracing failure as a natural part of the learning process, we can develop resilience, persistence, flexibility, positive thinking, and self-reflection skills that can help us to achieve our goals and reach our full potential.

How to Develop a Positive Attitude Towards Failure and How to Bounce Back From It

Developing a positive attitude towards failure can be challenging, but with some effort and practice, it is possible. Here are some strategies for developing a positive attitude towards failure and bouncing back from it:

Accept Failure as a Learning Opportunity: Rather than seeing failure as a negative experience, try to view it as an opportunity to learn and grow. Ask yourself what lessons you can take away from the experience and how you can use those lessons to improve in the future.

Practice Self-Compassion: It is important to be kind and compassionate towards yourself when you experience failure. Remember that everyone fails at some point, and that failure does not define your worth as a person. Treat yourself with the same kindness and understanding that you would offer to a friend who was going through a difficult time.

Focus on Your Strengths: When you experience failure, it can be easy to focus on your weaknesses or shortcomings. Instead, try to focus on your strengths and what you do well. This can help to boost your confidence and remind you of your abilities.

Set Realistic Goals: One of the reasons that failure can be so discouraging is that we often set unrealistic expectations for ourselves. When setting goals, try to make them challenging but realistic. This can help to increase your chances of success and reduce the likelihood of failure.

Develop a Growth Mindset: A growth mindset is the belief that intelligence and abilities can be developed over time through hard work and dedication. When you have a growth mindset, you are more likely to see failure as a temporary setback rather than a permanent obstacle.

Take Action: Finally, it is important to take action after experiencing failure. This might mean trying again with a new approach, seeking out feedback and advice from others, or simply taking some time to reflect and regroup. By taking action, you can regain a sense of control and momentum, which can help you to bounce back from failure and move forward towards your goals.

The Role of Confidence

Confidence plays a crucial role in taking risks because it helps us to believe in our abilities and make decisions with a sense of self-assurance. Here are some reasons why confidence is important in taking risks:

Confidence Boosts Self-Belief: When we have confidence, we are more likely to believe in ourselves and our abilities. This can be especially important when taking risks, as it can help us to trust our instincts and make bold decisions.

Confidence Helps to Overcome Fear: Taking risks can be scary, but having confidence can help us to push past our fears and take action despite the uncertainty. When we have confidence in our abilities, we are less likely to be held back by fear.

Confidence Increases Resilience: When we experience setbacks or failures, having confidence can help us to bounce back more quickly. With confidence, we are more likely to see failure as a temporary setback rather than a permanent obstacle.

Confidence Encourages Growth: When we take risks and step out of our comfort zones, we have the opportunity to learn and grow. With confidence, we are more likely to Accept these opportunities and see them as a chance to develop new skills and experiences.

Confidence Inspires Others: When we have confidence in ourselves and our abilities, we can inspire others to do the same. This can be especially important in professional settings, where confidence can help us to lead, motivate, and influence others.

Overall, having confidence is essential for taking risks and achieving success. While it can be challenging to build confidence, there are many strategies that can help, such as practicing self-care, setting achievable goals, and celebrating your successes along the way.

• Techniques for building self-belief, such as positive self-talk and visualization

Building self-belief is an important step in developing the confidence needed to take risks. Here are some techniques for building self-belief:

Practice Positive Self-Talk: The way we talk to ourselves can have a big impact on our self-belief. Try to challenge negative thoughts and replace them with positive affirmations. For example, instead of thinking "I'm not good enough," try replacing it with "I am capable and worthy of success."

Visualize Success: Visualization can be a powerful tool for building self-belief. Take some time to visualize yourself succeeding in your goals, and imagine the feelings of accomplishment and satisfaction that come with it.

Set Realistic Goals: Setting achievable goals and working towards them can help to build confidence and self-belief. Break your larger goals down into smaller, manageable steps, and celebrate each milestone along the way.

Seek Out Positive Feedback: Surround yourself with people who support and encourage you. Seek out constructive feedback from those you trust, and focus on the positive aspects of your progress and accomplishments.

Practice Self-Care: Taking care of yourself can help to build self-belief by promoting feelings of self-worth and confidence. Make sure to prioritize activities that make you feel good, such as exercise, meditation, or spending time with loved ones.

By incorporating these techniques into your daily routine, you can gradually build your self-belief and develop the confidence needed to take risks and achieve your goals. Remember that building self-belief takes time and effort, but with practice and persistence, you can develop a strong sense of self-confidence and belief in your abilities.

• The impact of self-confidence on success

Self-confidence is an essential ingredient for success. Here are some ways in which self-confidence impacts success:

Self-confidence allows you to take risks: When you have self-confidence, you are more willing to take risks and pursue opportunities that you might otherwise shy away from. This can lead to greater success in your personal and professional life.

Self-confidence helps you to overcome challenges: When faced with challenges or obstacles, self-confidence helps you to remain calm and focused, and to believe in your ability to overcome the challenge. This can help you to persevere through difficult times and come out stronger on the other side.

Self-confidence enhances your performance: When you believe in yourself, you are more likely to perform at your best. You are more likely to approach challenges with a positive attitude, and to put in the effort needed to achieve your goals.

Self-confidence helps you to communicate effectively: When you have self-confidence, you are more likely to communicate clearly and assertively, which can help you to build stronger relationships and achieve better outcomes in your personal and professional life.

Self-confidence promotes resilience: When you have self-confidence, you are better equipped to handle setbacks and failures. You are more likely to bounce back from adversity, and to see setbacks as opportunities for growth and learning.

Self-confidence plays a critical role in achieving success. By working to build your self-confidence through positive self-talk, visualization, and setting achievable goals, you can boost your chances of success in all areas of your life.

The Benefits of Risk-Taking Growth, Innovation, and Reward

• The rewards of taking risks, such as personal growth and innovation

Taking risks can lead to many rewards, including personal growth and innovation. Here are some ways in which taking risks can be beneficial:

Personal growth: When you take risks, you challenge yourself to step outside your comfort zone and try new things. This can lead to personal growth and development, as you gain new skills, knowledge, and experiences.

Innovation: Taking risks is often necessary to achieve innovation. By trying new approaches and ideas, you can discover new and better ways of doing things, which can lead to innovation and progress.

Increased confidence: Taking risks can help you to build self-confidence, as you prove to yourself that you are capable of taking on challenges and achieving your goals.

Greater resilience: Taking risks can also help you to develop resilience, as you learn to bounce back from setbacks and failures.

Career advancement: Taking risks can be beneficial for your career, as it can help you to stand out from others and demonstrate your willingness to take on challenges and pursue new opportunities.

In general, taking risks can be a powerful catalyst for personal and professional growth. By embracing risk-taking and being open to new challenges and opportunities, you can unlock your full potential and achieve greater success and fulfillment in your life.

• The relationship between risk-taking and achieving goals

Risk-taking and achieving goals are closely related, as taking risks can often be necessary to achieve one's goals. Here are some ways in which risk-taking can help you to achieve your goals:

Overcoming fear and uncertainty: Taking risks can help you to overcome fear and uncertainty, which can hold you back from pursuing your goals. By stepping outside your comfort zone and taking calculated risks, you can build confidence and develop the courage to pursue your goals.

Seizing opportunities: Opportunities often come with some level of risk. By being willing to take risks, you can seize opportunities that may otherwise be missed, and use them to achieve your goals.

Learning from failures: Taking risks also means accepting the possibility of failure. However, failure can be a valuable learning experience that can help you to grow and improve. By embracing risk-taking and learning from your failures, you can develop the resilience and determination needed to achieve your goals.

Pushing boundaries: Taking risks can help you to push the boundaries of what you thought was possible. By challenging yourself and taking on new challenges, you can achieve things that you may not have thought were possible.

Taking risks can be a powerful tool for achieving your goals. By being willing to take calculated risks, embracing uncertainty and failure, and seizing opportunities, you can unlock your full potential and achieve success in your personal and professional life.

• Identifying and measuring the benefits of taking risks

Taking risks can have many benefits, both in our personal and professional lives. Here are some of the benefits of taking risks:

Personal growth: Taking risks can help you to grow and develop as a person. By stepping outside your comfort zone and trying new things, you can build resilience, confidence, and self-belief.

Increased creativity and innovation: Taking risks can help you to think outside the box and come up with innovative ideas. By trying new things and exploring new possibilities, you can expand your creativity and find new solutions to old problems.

Improved decision-making skills: Taking risks requires careful analysis and evaluation of potential outcomes. By practicing risk-taking, you can improve your decision-making skills and learn how to weigh the pros and cons of different options.

Greater opportunities for success: Taking risks can open up new doors and create opportunities for success. By seizing opportunities that come with some level of risk, you can achieve things that you may not have thought possible.

Increased resilience: Taking risks involves accepting the possibility of failure. However, by embracing failure as a learning experience, you can develop resilience and the ability to bounce back from setbacks.

Measuring the benefits of taking risks can be difficult, as they are often intangible and subjective. However, by reflecting on your experiences and tracking your progress over time, you can begin to see the benefits of taking risks in your own life.

Identifying Opportunities

In 2007, the founders of Airbnb, Brian Chesky and Joe Gebbia, were struggling to pay their rent. With a design conference coming up in San Francisco, they decided to rent out air mattresses in their living room to conference attendees. After receiving positive feedback, they realized the potential of their idea and started Airbnb, a platform that allowed people to rent out their homes to travelers. Today, Airbnb is a billion-dollar company and has changed the way people travel.

In 2008, Travis Kalanick and Garrett Camp were attending a conference in Paris when they had trouble finding a taxi. This experience gave them the idea for Uber, a ride-hailing platform that connects drivers with riders. Despite initial resistance from traditional taxi companies and regulatory hurdles, Uber has become one of the most valuable companies in the world.

In 2010, four friends, Neil Blumenthal, Andrew Hunt, David Gilboa, and Jeffrey Raider, were frustrated with the high cost of eyeglasses. They started Warby Parker, an online eyeglasses retailer that offered affordable and stylish glasses. By cutting out the middleman and designing their own frames, they were able to offer high-quality glasses at a fraction of the cost of traditional retailers. Today, Warby Parker is valued at over $3 billion.

In the late 1990s, Sara Blakely was working as a salesperson and frustrated with the lack of comfortable and flattering undergarments. She came up with the idea for Spanx, a line of shapewear that smooths and slims the body. Despite being rejected by multiple manufacturers and retailers, Blakely persisted and launched Spanx in 2000. Today, Spanx is a multi-million dollar company and Blakely is one of the richest self-made women in the world.

All of these stories illustrate how individuals identified opportunities, took risks, and achieved success. By recognizing a need in the market and having the confidence to pursue their ideas, they were able to overcome obstacles and build successful businesses.

How to identify opportunities for taking risks

Identifying opportunities for taking risks can be challenging, as it requires a combination of creativity and strategic thinking. Here are some tips for identifying opportunities for taking risks:

Identify areas where you feel comfortable taking risks: Start by identifying areas in your personal or professional life where you feel comfortable taking risks. This might include areas where you have experience or expertise, or where you have a strong support system.

Look for opportunities to learn and grow: Seek out opportunities that challenge you and provide opportunities for growth and development. This might include taking on new projects or roles, or seeking out new experiences and opportunities outside your comfort zone.

Stay open to new possibilities: Be open to new ideas and opportunities that come your way, even if they initially seem outside your comfort zone. Sometimes the best opportunities for taking risks come from unexpected places.

Evaluate potential outcomes: When considering taking a risk, evaluate the potential outcomes and consider both the benefits and the risks. Think about what you have to gain and what you have to lose, and weigh these factors carefully.

Seek advice and support: Talk to friends, colleagues, or mentors who can provide guidance and support as you consider taking a risk. Their insights and perspectives can help you to make more informed decisions and minimize the potential for negative outcomes.

By staying open to new possibilities and carefully evaluating potential risks and benefits, you can identify opportunities for taking risks that can help you to achieve your goals and reach new heights of success and fulfillment.

Techniques for identifying potential risks and rewards

Here are some techniques for identifying potential risks and rewards associated with taking a particular action or decision:

Conduct a SWOT analysis: A SWOT analysis (Strengths, Weaknesses, Opportunities, Threats) is a useful tool for identifying potential risks and rewards associated with a particular course of action. This involves identifying the strengths and weaknesses of the decision, as well as any opportunities and threats that may arise.

Conduct a cost-benefit analysis: This technique involves weighing the potential costs and benefits associated with a decision or action. This helps you to understand the potential risks and rewards and make a more informed decision.

Evaluate past experiences: Reflecting on past experiences can help you to identify potential risks and rewards associated with similar decisions. This can help you to identify potential pitfalls and opportunities for success.

Seek advice and input from others: Talking to others who have experience or expertise in the area can help you to identify potential risks and rewards. This can provide a different perspective and help you to make a more informed decision.

Consider alternative scenarios: Thinking through alternative scenarios can help you to identify potential risks and rewards associated with different courses of action. This can help you to anticipate potential outcomes and make a more informed decision.

By using these techniques, you can identify potential risks and rewards associated with a particular decision or action. This can help you to make a more informed decision and minimize potential risks while maximizing potential rewards.

Recognizing The Potential For Growth

Recognizing the potential for growth is a crucial factor when considering taking risks. It is important to understand that taking risks can lead to new and unique experiences that can help an individual learn and grow. Some potential areas of growth that can be achieved through risk-taking include:

Personal growth: Taking risks can help an individual push beyond their comfort zone and learn more about themselves. They may discover new strengths, interests, or passions that they were previously unaware of.

Professional growth: Taking calculated risks can also lead to professional growth. It may help an individual develop new skills, gain new experiences, or open up new career opportunities.

Financial growth: In some cases, taking financial risks can lead to financial growth. For example, investing in a new business venture could potentially lead to significant financial rewards.

Relationship growth: Taking risks in relationships can also lead to growth. This can involve opening up about feelings, trying new activities together, or taking the next step in a relationship.

By recognizing the potential for growth, individuals can become more open to taking risks and embracing new experiences.

Developing a Risk-Taking Mindset

Developing a mindset that Accepts uncertainty is essential for individuals who wish to take risks. This involves accepting that the outcome of a risk is uncertain and being comfortable with that uncertainty. Here are some strategies for developing a mindset that Accepts uncertainty:

Reframe uncertainty: Rather than seeing uncertainty as a negative, reframe it as an opportunity. Uncertainty can bring excitement, creativity, and new possibilities.

Focus on the process, not just the outcome: When taking risks, it's important to focus on the journey, not just the end result. By enjoying the process, individuals can learn and grow, regardless of the outcome.

Practice mindfulness: Mindfulness can help individuals stay present in the moment and reduce anxiety about the future. This can be particularly helpful when taking risks, as it can help individuals stay focused and calm.

Accept failure: Failure is a natural part of taking risks, and it's important to Accept it as a learning opportunity. Rather than seeing failure as a setback, view it as a chance to learn and grow.

Surround yourself with support: Surrounding yourself with supportive people can help you stay positive and focused when taking risks. Seek out friends, family, or colleagues who will encourage and support you in your endeavors.

By developing a mindset that Accepts uncertainty, individuals can become more comfortable taking risks and more open to the possibilities that come with them.

Techniques For Overcoming Fear of The Unknown

Overcoming fear of the unknown is essential for taking risks and embracing uncertainty. Here are some techniques that can help:

Acceptance: Accept that the future is unknown and that there will always be some level of uncertainty in life.

Mindfulness: Practice mindfulness techniques to stay present in the moment and avoid getting caught up in anxious thoughts about the future.

Visualization: Visualize positive outcomes of taking risks and remind yourself of the potential rewards.

Education: Educate yourself about the risks and rewards of different options to help make informed decisions.

Planning: Plan for the worst-case scenario and have a backup plan in place.

Action: Take action to face your fears and take small steps towards embracing uncertainty.

Support: Surround yourself with supportive people who encourage you to take risks and help you overcome your fears.

Reflection: Reflect on past experiences where taking a risk paid off and remind yourself of your past successes.

By practicing these techniques, you can begin to overcome your fear of the unknown and develop a mindset that Accepts uncertainty.

The Impact of Mindset on Taking Risk

The impact of mindset on taking risks is significant. A growth mindset, which believes that abilities can be developed through dedication and hard work, is more likely to take risks than a fixed mindset, which believes that abilities are innate and cannot be changed.

When we adopt a growth mindset, we are more likely to see challenges as opportunities rather than obstacles. We are more likely to approach risk-taking with a sense of curiosity and a willingness to learn from our mistakes. This can lead to increased confidence and resilience, as we become more comfortable with uncertainty and are better equipped to handle setbacks.

On the other hand, a fixed mindset can lead us to view risks as threats rather than opportunities. We may feel that we are not capable of taking on new challenges or that failure is a reflection of our inherent limitations. This can lead to a fear of taking risks and a reluctance to step outside of our comfort zones.

For example, imagine two entrepreneurs who have developed a new product. One has a growth mindset and believes that if they work hard and take risks, they can achieve success. The other has a fixed mindset and believes that success is dependent on innate abilities, and taking risks is not worth it.

The entrepreneur with the growth mindset is more likely to take risks, such as investing money in marketing or expanding their product line, because they believe that hard work and dedication will lead to success. The entrepreneur with the fixed mindset, on the other hand, may be more cautious and less willing to take risks, as they believe that success is largely determined by innate abilities, and taking risks may not be worth the effort.

Therefore, developing a growth mindset can have a significant impact on one's willingness to take risks and ultimately, their success in life.

The Power of Persistence

Walt Disney, who faced numerous setbacks and failures before achieving success. Disney was fired from his job at a newspaper for lacking imagination and was told that his cartoons lacked marketability. He faced numerous business failures and even declared bankruptcy at one point.

However, Disney persisted and continued to pursue his vision of creating a theme park and producing feature-length animated films. His persistence paid off, and his company's creations, including Mickey Mouse, Snow White, and Disneyland, have become iconic symbols of American culture. Disney's story shows that even when facing seemingly insurmountable obstacles, persistence can help overcome setbacks and lead to great success.

• The importance of persistence in taking risks

Persistence is an essential trait when it comes to taking risks. It involves continuing to work towards a goal despite setbacks, failures, or challenges that may arise. Without persistence, it can be easy to give up on a goal or idea when faced with adversity, and risk-taking becomes less likely.

For example, let's say an entrepreneur wants to start a new business. They take a risk by investing a significant amount of time and money into the venture. However, things don't go as planned, and the business doesn't take off as quickly as expected. Without persistence, the entrepreneur might give up on the business and their goal of running a successful company.

On the other hand, if the entrepreneur is persistent, they will continue to work towards their goal, even if it means making changes to their business strategy or seeking help from others. Over time, their persistence can pay off, and they may be able to achieve success in their venture.

Therefore, persistence is crucial for taking risks because it helps individuals stay committed to their goals despite obstacles and setbacks. Without it, risk-taking becomes less effective, and the potential for success is diminished.

• Techniques for overcoming setbacks and obstacles

When taking risks, setbacks and obstacles are common. Therefore, it is essential to develop techniques for overcoming them. Here are some techniques for overcoming setbacks and obstacles:

Reframe your perspective: Instead of viewing setbacks as failures, try to reframe them as opportunities to learn and grow. This shift in perspective can help you approach setbacks with a growth mindset.

Practice self-compassion: Be kind to yourself when facing setbacks. Remember that setbacks are a natural part of the risk-taking process, and it is normal to feel disappointed or frustrated. Practice self-compassion by acknowledging your emotions and giving yourself permission to feel them.

Break down the problem: When faced with a complex problem, it can be helpful to break it down into smaller, more manageable parts. This approach can help you identify the root cause of the problem and develop a more effective solution.

Seek feedback: Getting feedback from others can provide valuable insight into how to overcome setbacks and obstacles. Seek out mentors or peers who can offer constructive feedback and guidance.

Keep moving forward: Finally, it is essential to keep moving forward, even in the face of setbacks. Persistence is key to achieving success, and setbacks should not deter you from continuing to pursue your goals. Every failure is an opportunity to learn and grow, and use these experiences to fuel your persistence and determination.

How to Develop a Positive Attitude

Developing a positive attitude towards challenges and adversity is essential for overcoming obstacles and achieving success. Here are some techniques that can help:

Reframe your mindset: Instead of seeing challenges and adversity as negative events, try to see them as opportunities for growth and development. This can help you approach them with a positive and proactive attitude.

Focus on solutions: Rather than dwelling on the problem or obstacle, shift your focus to finding solutions. Ask yourself, "What can I do to overcome this challenge?" or "What steps can I take to move forward?"

Practice self-compassion: Be kind and compassionate towards yourself, especially during difficult times. Remind yourself that everyone faces challenges and setbacks, and that it's okay to make mistakes or fall short of your goals.

Accept failure: Instead of fearing failure, Accept it as a necessary part of the learning process. Use your failures as opportunities to learn, grow, and improve.

Set realistic expectations: When facing a challenge or adversity, it's important to set realistic expectations for yourself. This can help you avoid becoming overwhelmed or discouraged.

Seek support: Don't be afraid to reach out to friends, family, or a professional for support during challenging times. Having a support system can help you stay positive and motivated.

Conclusion

In conclusion, taking risks is a crucial aspect of personal and professional growth. The book *"The Art of Taking Risks"* provides an insightful and informative perspective on how to take calculated risks and make informed decisions.

The book emphasizes the importance of considering the potential costs and drawbacks of taking a risk, along with the potential benefits. By assessing the level of risk, the individual can determine if the potential benefits outweigh the potential costs, and if the risk is worth taking.

Furthermore, the book stresses the importance of aligning risks with personal values and goals. Taking a risk that aligns with personal values can provide a sense of purpose and meaning, which ultimately leads to greater satisfaction and success.

The author also emphasizes the importance of intuition in decision making. While weighing the potential risks and benefits logically is crucial, one should not ignore their intuition. Listening to one's intuition can provide a unique perspective and help in making an informed decision.

Moreover, the book highlights the importance of developing abilities and acquiring necessary resources to handle potential risks and challenges. This is an important step in making informed decisions and reducing the chances of failure.

The author emphasizes the importance of having a support system. Taking risks can be challenging, and having a support system can help provide guidance and support during tough times.

Overall, "*The Art of Taking Risks*" is an informative and insightful book that provides an excellent framework for making informed decisions and taking calculated risks. By considering the potential benefits and costs, aligning risks with personal values and goals, and having a support system in place, individuals can take risks with greater confidence and ultimately achieve greater success.

In today's world, where rapid technological advancements, economic uncertainties, and changing social norms have made life unpredictable, taking risks has become more important than ever. This book will be a valuable resource for anyone seeking to take risks, achieve personal or professional growth, and ultimately live a fulfilling life.

Well done on finishing the book "The Art of taking Risk". Now, take a moment to assess your risk taking ability:-

Instructions:

1. For each question, select the option that best reflects your feelings or behaviors.
2. Choose only one option per question.
3. Be honest in your responses to get an accurate assessment of your risk-taking capability.
4. Assign points on a scale of 1 to 5, where 1 indicates the least agreement and 5 indicates the highest agreement.

Questions:

1. **I am comfortable with uncertainty and ambiguity.**

   a. Strongly Agree (5)

   b. Agree (4)

   c. Neutral (3)

   d. Disagree (2)

   e. Strongly Disagree (1)

2. **I often seek out new and challenging experiences.**

   a. Strongly Agree (5)

   b. Agree (4)

   c. Neutral (3)

   d. Disagree (2)

   e. Strongly Disagree (1)

3. **I see failures as opportunities for learning and growth.**

   a. Strongly Agree (5)

b. Agree (4)

c. Neutral (3)

d. Disagree (2)

e. Strongly Disagree (1)

4. **I am willing to take risks even if the outcome is uncertain.**

a. Strongly Agree (5)

b. Agree (4)

c. Neutral (3)

d. Disagree (2)

e. Strongly Disagree (1)

5. **I enjoy stepping out of my comfort zone to explore new possibilities.**

a. Strongly Agree (5)

b. Agree (4)

c. Neutral (3)

d. Disagree (2)

e. Strongly Disagree (1)

6. **I often challenge the status quo and conventional thinking.**

a. Strongly Agree (5)

b. Agree (4)

c. Neutral (3)

d. Disagree (2)

e. Strongly Disagree (1)

7. **I take calculated risks in my personal and professional life.**

a. Strongly Agree (5)

b. Agree (4)

c. Neutral (3)

d. Disagree (2)

e. Strongly Disagree (1)

8. **I am open to feedback and constructive criticism even if it involves risk.**

a. Strongly Agree (5)

b. Agree (4)

c. Neutral (3)

d. Disagree (2)

e. Strongly Disagree (1)

9. **I believe in my ability to overcome challenges and setbacks.**

a. Strongly Agree (5)

b. Agree (4)

c. Neutral (3)

d. Disagree (2)

e. Strongly Disagree (1)

10. **I am comfortable making decisions without all the information.**

a. Strongly Agree (5)

b. Agree (4)

c. Neutral (3)

d. Disagree (2)

e. Strongly Disagree (1)

11. **I am drawn to opportunities that involve risk rather than sticking to the safe path.**

a. Strongly Agree (5)

b. Agree (4)

c. Neutral (3)

d. Disagree (2)

e. Strongly Disagree (1)

12. **I often find myself taking risks in pursuit of my goals and aspirations.**

a. Strongly Agree (5)

b. Agree (4)

c. Neutral (3)

d. Disagree (2)

e. Strongly Disagree (1)

13. **I enjoy the thrill and excitement that come with taking risks.**

a. Strongly Agree (5)

b. Agree (4)

c. Neutral (3)

d. Disagree (2)

e. Strongly Disagree (1)

14. **I believe that taking risks is essential for personal and professional development.**

a. Strongly Agree (5)

b. Agree (4)

c. Neutral (3)

d. Disagree (2)

e. Strongly Disagree (1)

15. **I have a high tolerance for ambiguity and unforeseen challenges.**

a. Strongly Agree (5)

b. Agree (4)

c. Neutral (3)

d. Disagree (2)

e. Strongly Disagree (1)

16. **I feel comfortable making decisions that may have uncertain outcomes.**

a. Strongly Agree (5)

b. Agree (4)

c. Neutral (3)

d. Disagree (2)

e. Strongly Disagree (1)

17. **I actively seek out opportunities to take risks in my daily life.**

a. Strongly Agree (5)

b. Agree (4)

c. Neutral (3)

d. Disagree (2)

e. Strongly Disagree (1)

18. **I believe that avoiding all risks can hinder personal and professional growth.**

a. Strongly Agree (5)

b. Agree (4)

c. Neutral (3)

d. Disagree (2)

e. Strongly Disagree (1)

19. **I find excitement in situations where the outcome is uncertain.**

a. Strongly Agree (5)

b. Agree (4)

c. Neutral (3)

d. Disagree (2)

e. Strongly Disagree (1)

20. **I am willing to take risks for the sake of innovation and progress.**

a. Strongly Agree (5)

b. Agree (4)

c. Neutral (3)

d. Disagree (2)

e. Strongly Disagree (1)

21. **I am open to exploring opportunities that may involve a level of risk.**

a. Strongly Agree (5)

b. Agree (4)

c. Neutral (3)

d. Disagree (2)

e. Strongly Disagree (1)

22. **I view uncertainty as a potential for positive change and growth.**

a. Strongly Agree (5)

b. Agree (4)

c. Neutral (3)

d. Disagree (2)

e. Strongly Disagree (1)

23. **I am comfortable with making decisions that challenge the status quo.**

a. Strongly Agree (5)

b. Agree (4)

c. Neutral (3)

d. Disagree (2)

e. Strongly Disagree (1)

24.   **I am willing to take risks even if it means stepping into the unknown.**

a. Strongly Agree (5)

b. Agree (4)

c. Neutral (3)

d. Disagree (2)

e. Strongly Disagree (1)

25.   **I believe that risk-taking is an integral part of personal success.**

a. Strongly Agree (5)

b. Agree (4)

c. Neutral (3)

d. Disagree (2)

e. Strongly Disagree (1)

26.   **I often find myself seeking out opportunities that involve a degree of risk.**

a. Strongly Agree (5)

b. Agree (4)

c. Neutral (3)

d. Disagree (2)

e. Strongly Disagree (1)

27.   **I am open to making decisions that may go against conventional wisdom.**

a. Strongly Agree (5)

b. Agree (4)

c. Neutral (3)

d. Disagree (2)

e. Strongly Disagree (1)

28.   **I am comfortable making choices that others might perceive as risky.**

a. Strongly Agree (5)

b. Agree (4)

c. Neutral (3)

d. Disagree (2)

e. Strongly Disagree (1)

29. **I am willing to face challenges head-on even if it involves taking risks.**

a. Strongly Agree (5)

b. Agree (4)

c. Neutral (3)

d. Disagree (2)

e. Strongly Disagree (1)

30. **I believe that risk-taking is necessary for achieving personal fulfillment.**

a. Strongly Agree (5)

b. Agree (4)

c. Neutral (3)

d. Disagree (2)

e. Strongly Disagree (1)

Scoring:

Add up the points for each response. The total score will reflect your overall risk-taking capability.

Join My Community

https://community.askpndas.com/

The other books in the series, 'The Art of Living